April
is Not Always
The Cruelest Month

Twenty-one days of focused writing

Terry Crawford Palardy

ISBN: **13: 978-1523332786**
: 1523332786

DEDICATION

*Always dedicated to
my husband
my best friend
my coach
my partner
and my love, Rick*

ACKNOWLEDGMENT

*I was inspired and guided in this writing endeavor by the **WEGO Health Social Network's** Writing Prompts for April, 2012, to which I responded in my blog, http://Terry'sThoughtsandThreads.blogspot.com This book contains some of those blog entries.*

1

***Imagine what you might put into
a health time-capsule to be opened
one hundred years from today.***

"What do you think it is?"
"I don't know yet ... I can't get it open, it's covered in tape. It must have been up here in the rafters of this old barn for decades."
"Maybe it's a deed ... or a certificate of stock ... maybe it's something really valuable! Hurry up, open it!"
"Let me get one of those old tools we saw below, the one with the plastic handle and the flat end on the rod..."

The two brothers jumped down the short distance from the attic of their great-grandfather's barn. The tool they found was encrusted in rust and of no use to them, so they took they small packet into the house, where they placed it on the chopping block table. Reaching for a pair of zip scissors, they sliced off a sixteenth of an inch from one edge, and reached inside. The page inside was neatly creased and fell into two sections when unfolded.

"It's a letter, dated 2012, and signed by our great-great-great-grandmother! Remember the story of the package of pages tied in ribbons that our great grandmother found about fifty years ago, the one that told all about life at the turn of the millennium? She gave it to the historical society when she found it. Dad told me that his grandmother wanted people to know what life was like for women born in the twentieth century. The pages were all about school-teaching, and learning to use primitive technology by typing on a keyboard ..."

"Read it! Why did she leave this note out in the barn? Why wasn't it with the rest of the pages? Is it really from her? Is it really a hundred years old? How old was she when she wrote it?"

"Give me a minute ... this one is hand-written, in the old style, with the loopy letters, and the ink is fading. Here's what I think it says:"

For whoever finds this note, please excuse the handwriting. My eyesight is worsening and the tremors in my hands are increasing, but I wanted to write this with liquid ink, so that it wouldn't fade away as print might.

They tell me I have multiple sclerosis. I don't really believe them, for no one in my family, for generations past, has ever been labeled such. My father, his brother, and his mother all had Parkinson's Disease, and they showed the same symptoms that I have. But the doctors who diagnosed me disregard that history, for doctors in the past hadn't the modern technology of magnetic resonance imaging that we have. The clunking, banging, noisy scans reveal innumerable lesions on my brain, and on my spine. And the lumbar puncture, the long needle poked into my spinal cord, revealed bands in my spinal fluid, and that too is said to be an indicator of MS.

My first neurologist insisted on ruling everything else out, and said that I didn't have PD because my arms did not jerk when he rotated my elbow. He prescribed what was thought to be important: a disease modifying drug that I would have to inject with a syringe every night, rotating among seven different areas of my body that had adequate layers of fat beneath the skin. Just the thought of that annoyed me, but he said that it would possibly delay the progression of multiple sclerosis' nerve degeneration by about a third. Small promise, I thought. But I went along with his prescription.

For almost five years I and my husband patiently, carefully, scheduled and rotated the injections, which always burned for twenty minutes afterward. But when I began to read about differences of opinion regarding the cause of this so-far incurable disease, and read that some disagreed that it was an immune disorder, seeing it rather as a metabolic disorder, I knew that my choice at diagnosis to change my eating style was a good decision, and was probably enough. No meat, no dairy products other than yogurt, nothing fried ... I'd lost a good deal of weight that first year, and hadn't had a relapse since diagnosis.

Oh, I'd had symptoms, but they were never called relapses. In my late fifties, a cataract could be causing the blurred vision. Weakness and vertigo in the hot humid summer was attributed to the weather, as it could be easily remedied by moving into a cooler space. Depression, anxiety and fear, loss of the ability to learn new things by reading, and forgetting my students' names were all attributed to life stresses. I had to leave my beloved classroom, and retire a few years earlier than planned.

When that happened to me, I made my decision to discontinue the injections, and soon felt more like myself. My energy increased, my ability to read and write improved, and without the stress of the classroom and with antidepressant medication, I began to take an interest in life again. It was too late to save my teaching career, and my ability to remember new things was never going to return to what it had been when I could learn one hundred new student names and profiles every year, but I could begin a new career.

And that is why I'm writing today. I want to tell my children's children, and their grandchildren's grandchildren, to listen to their inner selves. I want to show them that taking care of their metabolism is important. I want them to know that eating a menu of vegetables, beans, seeds, and berries is a healthy choice. I want them to recognize that when a medication with slim promises doesn't help and causes more issues than existed before it is okay to tell a doctor 'No thank you.'

I suppose in a few more decades, or half a century ahead, or in the next century itself, all of this will seem primitive and ridiculous. When we look back at how illness was treated a century ago, in 1912, when people with Parkinson's Disease or assumed Multiple Sclerosis were told simply to go home and rest, limiting their strength by inactivity, we shake our heads and say they ought to have known better.

Perhaps my descendents will look upon today's medical advancements as short-sighted. Maybe the nutritional aspects of disease symptoms will be looked at first in the next century. We look back today at the twentieth century's widespread use of pesticides and herbicides and shake our heads, realizing the damage they have caused to ourselves and to our gene pools.

At any rate, whoever is reading this: you have the opportunity and responsibility to live a healthier lifestyle. We began to make forward steps at the beginning of this twenty-first century. We recognized the faults of the earlier generations, and did our best to avoid the known carcinogens in our environments and in our lifestyle choices.

Know that I love you, and want the best for you.
It is up to you to seek it out.
Terry Crawford Palardy

PS: I asked my husband to tuck this note into the rafters of the barn because, as anyone alive today knows, the barns are often kept in better shape than the houses, for it is the barns that allow a space to earn a living.

"Wow. It really is her note. She could be standing right here, talking to us."

"What are we going to do with this? Give it to the historical society? They can add it to the database and store it away with her other writings."

"I guess so. I don't know, it seems like something we ought to share with someone ... but who?"

The boys left the packet on the table, planning to show it to their dad, later.

2

**_Choose a quote that inspires you
(positively or negatively)
and free-write about it._**

_"Our most basic common link is that we
all inhabit this planet. We all breathe
the same air. We all cherish our
children's future. And we are all
mortal." JFK_

Common links ... breathing the same air ...
cherishing children ... cherishing their future ...
recognizing mortality. I had this quote on a large
poster of John Fitzgerald Kennedy, and hung it on
the corridor wall outside my classroom. When I
retired, I found a friend in the building that shared
my admiration of this president, and who would
promise to use the poster well.

Kennedy was our president at the end of the Happy Days of the 1950s. He inherited the worries of a conflicted world across a different ocean, the Pacific. Vietnam was still being viewed as just a conflict, a place for America to step in and advise struggling countries. The cold war between America and the former USSR was well established, and the enemy was communism (or, to the other side, capitalism.)

It was easy for JFK to impress me, as I was a ten year old when he was elected president. He was my president; I campaigned for him, carrying a homemade sign carefully lettered and spelled correctly, and I celebrated when he won the election despite the obvious handicaps ... being another from Boston ... being Catholic in a time when domination from across the seas was a threat to many, whether it might come from Russia or from Rome.

JFK had young children. He had a beautiful wife. He had experience in the World War, and was a hero before he was president. His family came from the same city that I came from. He was from a family as large as my own. How could I not admire him?

When I was an adult, and he was long gone, the scandals were dragged out of the family closet. His beautiful wife went on to another marriage, in another country, and moved in even higher circles than she had as a young political wife. She became a symbol for all of the American women who lost husbands and fiancés and brothers in the Vietnam "Conflict." But living as a symbol when the reason for your symbolism is removed was perhaps more than she would choose, and she moved on with her life.

JFK knew that we were all mortal. He knew that we needed to protect the air that we all breathed, in an era when countries were competing with each other to have the most powerful and destructive tools of war. But he believed in a better use of scientific knowledge, and he authorized two vastly different programs: the race for the moon, and the Peace Corps. Because he did, man looked outward to the heavens and wondered about life beyond our atmosphere, and we began to look within our own sphere and recognize that things here needed more protection, more appreciation, and more collaboration.

It is not only because I was ten and easily inspired: JFK was the right man for our world at the time we all knew him. How sad that when he was gone, the appreciation was not sustained. We grew up, and are now older than he ever had a chance to be. In honor of his goals, and in respect for his memory, we all must do the best we can to protect this air that we all breathe, and to continue to cherish our children's future.

3

If you had a superpower, what would it be and how would you use it?

Hmmm ... a superpower. What would it be? What would I most like to have as a superpower? And if I did use it, would it benefit some without causing harm to others?

For example, mind-reading ... if I could read others' minds, recognizing truth vs lies, courage vs bravado, honesty vs deception ... what would I do with that knowledge? Would I make my power known publicly, as Superman did? Or would I hide my power from others to protect myself from those seeking power over others? Would I be so distracted by others' thoughts that I would lose awareness of my own? Or would I use that knowledge to try to intercede in conflicts about to be, in the optimistic belief that I could make a difference if only I knew what motivated the disagreements ... or would that intervention serve only to make things worse?

Or would I want a superpower that was physically beneficial? If I suddenly became invincibly strong, able to lift great weights, or dive to great depths, or climb mountains tirelessly, or run endlessly at great speeds... perhaps that strength would have value a hundred years ago, but technology today can help people do all of that virtually, communally, through immediate technological communications, explorations, and demonstrations.

Could I have a superpower that would make a difference in the world's political arena? If I were able to implant positive, peaceful motivations in world leaders' minds leading to the recognition that, regardless of geographic location or economic situations we ought to act as one united human race, protecting our planet from further devastation, pollution, and consumption? Would my priorities, my beliefs, my values and my humility and altruistic desires serve to better the human race's situation? Could I make the best decisions?

If I had a superpower in my brain, a creative discovery of the best way to grow enough crops in even the worst climates and soils, to help every area on earth become self-sustaining and not dependent, would it allow various cultures to retain their identities without retaining their legacies of hardship, starvation and disease? Could such a brain recognize and share natural disease treatments? Would the population then increase exponentially across the globe? How many years would the natural resources last? Would a super-powered brain be able to plan for that?

I'm not a super-powered being. I'm a rational
American, one who has followed the rules, set goals,
and worked toward them, accomplishing much
along the way and learning to accept the shortfalls
that come with life. I think often of the word
Namaste ... translated by Mother Teresa to "I see
God in every human being" and by the people of
Hindu belief as "I recognize and bow to the divine in
you, as you do in me." If we all could accept that
premise of life, what a beautiful race we could be,
with the superpower of respect.

4

Why do I write about my health? The answer
to that question has changed through the years, as
has my health.

In the years prior to diagnosis, I wrote more about
my parents' health. They both experienced difficult
health issues during the last two decades of their
lives: a pacemaker for one, a new hip for the other,
failing eyesight with age, cancer surgery for both,
and then Alzheimer's and Parkinson's. I kept track
of their symptoms, prescriptions, appointments
(with my husband's help) ... I was their health
proxy, and so I was in contact with their doctors
(with my sister's help) ... and what symptoms I had
myself took a back seat until their issues brought
closure to their lives.

And then I wrote of my symptoms, fully expecting to
follow my parents' path toward Parkinson's Disease.
But along the way diagnostic tests, appointments,
doctors' names and my own health proxy (my

husband) became the topics in my journal. The completion of those tests led to the diagnosis of relapsing remitting multiple sclerosis. It was not what I'd anticipated, but it was what I got. And with it, I was given a prescription for a disease modifying drug, but no cure.

My journal entries darkened with anger, and trembled with frustration, anxiety, and fear. How could I have multiple sclerosis? No one I knew had ever had this diagnosis. How could I give myself an injection each night? How could I ask my husband, who had managed his own parents' illnesses, involving cancer, blindness, COPD and depression, as well as assisting with all my parents' care ... how could I ask him now to help me? How could I go into my classroom each day for another six years, and finish my career on my feet, with the dignity I'd worked so hard to preserve?

My writing helped me to realize that my disagreement with this diagnosis might be disputed by scientific evidence ... the lesions were there ... but my inner self believed that the diagnosis was wrong, and so the treatment was wrong. It was horribly expensive, and though I had a good insurance policy and paid only a small fraction of the thousands of dollars it cost each month, I knew that policy holders' premiums were going up each year, as was the price of my medication. I felt it was unnecessary; I felt it was wrong; I feared that, if it was wrong, it could be causing more damage rather than repairing anything. It made only vague promises of perhaps slowing the progression by 30%, but no guarantee for any one patient. And it interacted with my immune system, which worried me.

I was experiencing no relapses, but I attributed that to my change in menu and my loss of fifty excess pounds, the resulting lowered blood pressure and better energy levels. But through the four and a half years of this treatment, I became more depressed and more fearful of what it might be doing, and writing out those fears, and explaining with written words those disagreements and my rationale for them, I was able to make the decision to follow my heart and discontinue the treatments.

Had I not written my story, I may not have had the courage to follow my beliefs. I am no longer taking the injections with their prohibitive financial costs … I no longer feel like a fraud carrying a diagnosis that didn't seem real, and I am feeling better each day. I recently walked five miles to raise money for MS research, and I have no reason to stop doing that.

Some say my feeling better is simply a placebo effect; I want to believe that I am better without the injections, and so I believe I am feeling better. But I say perhaps it was my own belief that the medication was doing me harms that made me weaken while taking it, and so not taking it has relieved that burden of worry, depression and anxiety that I had taken on myself. Who is to say whether they or I am right or wrong?

The experts in the study of multiple sclerosis are also conflicted; the assumption that treating the immune system will slow the progression is now being disputed not just by patients like me, but by doctors who are saying this may be a metabolic issue rather than an immune disorder; it may be related to the nutrients needed for healthy mitochondria, in which case my healthier diet was the right choice to make, and that is a validating statement for me. Vitamin D is finally being discussed more openly rather than being left unaddressed.

I will stay in the seven year Parkinson's Disease risk study with the National Institute of Health in Bethesda, if they will have me. There is some question as to whether my current prescription of anti-depressant will conflict with their protocol of testing, and so I may not be able to participate until I have been able to stop that medication. I will write about that in the weeks to come. If I am in their study group, their testing will show any indicators of Parkinson's Disease earlier than might be known if not in the study group. And contrary as it sounds, that medication treatment is one I would willingly take, in an effort to study its efficacy and benefit future generations of my family, and beyond.

I will continue to walk for MS, because I can. And in time I will begin to walk for Parkinson's Disease fundraising, for as long as I can. I still believe that is what lies ahead in my future. The tremors that I experience resemble those of my mother and father. Time will be the judge of whether that, too, is right or wrong.

5

Go to flickr.com and write a post inspired by the image... link it to your health focus.

I found at that page Rodin's sculpture, **The Farewell**. and wrote what elicited this initial reaction/post from me:

The eyes appear to be looking to the left, indicating a memory. The hands seem to be repressing a spoken thought, remembering something that ought not be shared. It's a pensive pose, and one suggesting some confusion. The word "enigma" is titling the post of this image.

I use the word enigma in my book title, Multiple Sclerosis an Enigma. It is a diagnosis that leaves one with only unknowns, and regrets for having sought an answer but having found only more questions. I was my doctor's enigma, a patient with a great deal of clinical evidence of the disease but showing few visible symptoms, and no acceptance of what science pronounced as true.

I've often written in my journal of the losses brought to me with this diagnosis. My reaction to the treatment prescribed was negative, prompting unwanted feelings of present and future losses, beginning with the loss of energy (fatigue), organizational skills (depression related) and anxiety (also depression related.) These losses led to the loss of my career (public school teacher) and my self-image (30 years of successful teaching and collegiality.) My loss of my classroom created a void in my social contacts, loss of my partners and their wit and wisdom. I might well have, at times, taken the pose of Rodin's sculpture.

But that was in the past, and the present is better.

6
Write a haiku about health

Haiku is a 5-7-5 poem. Haiku's are generally about nature, with a final line that leaves a lasting image with the reader (or listener.)

I am sitting here, wondering how to link the themes of nature and health. It will not be hard, healthy choices are all part of our natural world. If I do it right, it will offer positive wisdom you can keep.

Writing a Haiku takes a little planning but will be worth the time. Holding to just three lines of nature's symmetry: that will be our task. It need not be hard; nature offers so many patterns we can view. Make the healthy choice, share in Nature's abundance and reap the rewards!

I am sitting here,
wondering how to link the themes
of nature and health.

It will not be hard,
healthy choices are all part

of our natural world.

If I do it right,
it will offer positive
wisdom you can keep .

Writing a Haiku
takes a little planning but
will be worth the time.

Holding to just three
lines of nature's symmetry
that will be our task

It need not be hard,
nature offers so many
patterns we can view.

Make the healthy choice

Share in her abundance

And reap her rewards.

7

Write about What You Want Today.

I thought I was on track for securing what I want. I had gone to college because my guidance counselor saw potential in me. When I finished the two-year school, I headed into the work force, and then married, and began a family, which is what I'd wanted to do. And I was happy.

The economy, though, was crashing in the early seventies; gas was rationed to every other day purchasing, inflation was eating up what I could earn in my part time position in a department store that was seeing a slowdown of purchasing, and I realized that the time had come to go back to college while it was still affordable and get that teaching degree that would let me take a stable position. That was the new want - I wanted to teach, and to work in a secure environment that would not be harmed by fluctuations in the stock market and in supply and demand. There would always be a demand for teachers, for there would always be students. And when I finally signed the teaching contract six years later, I was happy.

Our family continued to grow, first with a second child, and then with grandchildren. It grew and grew with cousins, and we often got together to share holidays. But then it began to shrink: our parents were aging and declining, and needing more help from us. When they had finished passing through the sadness of decline, and were laid to rest, I looked at where we were then, saw that I had managed to keep my job and my professional reputation intact, and saw that we still had each other, and I was happy.

When my own symptoms took me to the doctors' offices, and I learned that they believed I had multiple sclerosis, I decided to comply with the diagnosis and take the prescribed injections each night, rather than taking the less frequent interferons which could have interrupted my attendance at school. I stuck with that prescription for four and a half years, following it downward into a depression so deep that I needed additional doctors and prescriptions to help me out of it. When I finally exited that, I decided to go with my inner belief and stop the injections, as their side effects of depression and anxiety had already cost me my teaching position. With the guidance of family and friends, I got through the paperwork and secured a pension; it was less than it would have been had I been able to stay longer, but what happened had happened, and was irreversible. I once again took stock: I realized I had completed thirty years in the classrooms, believed I had done some good, and still had a happy marriage and so I could be happy about that.

So, what do I want today? I'd like to say I know what I want, and that I have a plan. Truth be told, I am happy with the way things evolved thus far. It would be nice to earn a little extra money to compensate for the shortfall in my pension, but in time, we will have some of the larger bills paid off: bills I took on believing I would have two more years of full salary to pay for them, but I haven't, and so we're tightening out belt until they are paid.

I don't want for much, ever. My father told me years ago, when he retired, that we didn't have much, but we had enough. It is my mantra now. There isn't much left to want; I have it all. Peace, love, a home, food to eat, and a family with which to share my stories. It is enough.

8

"Best conversation I had this week."

I had an online conversation with a woman who found me on Facebook: she is a cousin going back in my maternal grandmother's family line.

The day she contacted me was my mother's birthday, and the name that caught her eye was my mother's maiden name: Buxey. My name then is only a few degrees removed from her own; her maternal grandfather was my grandmother's first cousin.

After ascertaining that I was related to her, she offered to send the information on her branch of the family, and offered me another Facebook contact: that of a retired genealogist in South Africa, who has traced the Buxey family back as far as 1616 in England. This is a branch of our family about which I knew very little. I knew that my grandmother's grandmother had come from county Tyrone, Ireland, had lost her husband on the voyage over, and had then married a young British officer supervising the immigration. Beyond that, information was sketchy at best.

My parents had sat with relatives in the late 1960's to begin to draw up a chart of ancestors this side of the Atlantic. I have a few small pieces of paper written by my father's sister, giving the names of his mother and her brothers who emigrated from Edinburgh and Leith in Scotland, and the larger piece of paper in my parents' hand-writings listing the parents and grandparents of both sides of the family. But in the larger scheme, my mother's information showed only a small portion of her mother's family.

Her mother was one of twelve sisters and brothers, and the information given to me this week shows the descendents of many of those many relatives. With today's internet access, reaching out to a far removed cousin in South Africa seems natural, and common. I've forwarded the information that I gained on to my own sisters and brother, and my mother's nieces and nephews, all of whom will expand our family's branch of this developing lineage.

The history teacher within me marvels at the Canadian great-grandparents who were born just before and just after America's Civil War Period, and those names recorded in church papers in England during the Protestant Reformation almost five hundred years ago. It is the family treasure that will be passed on to our own descendants, and one that we might never have known were it not for the internet connections of today. Whatever roles relatives may or may not have played in history's tableau remains to be discovered.

There was a family Bible begun with my parents' wedding in 1940, and it rests with one of my sisters now ... perhaps this new information will be placed within its covers in time. Meanwhile, it is still my intention to continue recording my own portion of the timeline, at the website titled Beyond Old Windows, and in packets of year by year pages tied in ribbons for my one day great-great-great grandchildren to find, and to share.

9

Keep Calm and Carry On

That's a tall order: keep calm and carry on. Yet it is what most of us do instinctively. One foot in front of the other, head down to watch where the steps may lead, don't try to walk and chew gum at the same time ...

It also helps to look back and see what you have already been through; you have probably faced many, varied challenges in life, and each time it may have seemed impossibly complex and dangerously strong, yet you are here today. You made it through that very dark time, over those incredible hurdles, in the face of such powerful self-doubt.

It does also help to look ahead now and then, to ascertain that you are indeed on a path that will lead to something. Setting goals gets a lot of talk-time in schools, and aiming high (even higher than may be conceivable) is encouraged. Applying to ten or twelve colleges seems excessive in some high schools and barely adequate in others, and waiting for the responses can seem excruciatingly silent for a period of weeks or months, but most students do survive the passage from high school on to further academia or technical training.

My take on all of that is to stay focused on where you are right now, and make it the best that it can be. While you are looking back at dark times overcome, and while you are looking ahead to scope out the future passage, don't miss the view of now. Take it all in. What is working for you, or against you, right now? What can realistically be done to alter it, better it, or banish it? How can you move forward? Is forward the right direction? Is up always better? Trains circle and loop to gain altitude on a mountain; others tunnel right through the depths. Can an obstacle in your path be circumvented rather than overcome? Is right always best?

And when does pace come into the equation? Must you go to college right away? Would a year or two of employment enhance your understanding of what your goals may be? Would it add to or deplete savings you set aside for education? Is what you could be doing right now as valuable as education?

My dad told me once, as I was fretting over a conflict in goals between myself and the new administrator appointed above my position who had totally different goals and experiences, that if I am facing a stone wall, impenetrable, and too steep to climb despite my best efforts, I perhaps would do better by turning away from the wall, and moving in a different direction, one which might lead me to some place where my energy would be well spent , where I could do good, and succeed, and help others to succeed. It's good to have a Plan B in your pocket. It's good to notice what else you might be good at, what else the 'now' has been preparing you for, in case your path leads to a goal erased.

Einstein, Edison, and correspondent Peter Jennings reached success and notoriety by taking alternate paths: Einstein was not your standardized student; Edison learned by making mistake after mistake, and Jennings skipped academia for work experience. Surely their paths had challenges, and were frowned upon by the establishment. But they found their path to success. They followed it where it took them, and I believed they paid attention to the now around them, always, while getting from past to future.

Keeping calm is easier if you believe that you are heading in the right direction, acquiring the right skills, finding the right supports and mentors, and an adequate amount of time to practice and observe results before moving on. People need to remember the old Apple IIe computer: while uploading a quantity of graphic data, there was a pause before downloading it to the printer. Apple's screen would flash the words "Thinking, thinking, thinking"... before then flashing "Printing, printing, printing" and then returning to repeat the cycle in order to carry on with the rest of the data. Such a valuable lesson. Such a calm, confident example.

10

Write a Letter to 16-year-old-me

April 10, 2012

Dear 16-year-old-me,

I'm writing this from your future, and I know all
that lies ahead for you on this path. You are a junior
in high school right now, and it is the year 1966.
Your greatest fear is that your friend Rick, your soon
to be fiancé, will be drafted when he finishes school.
Many who don't go on to college go instead to the
'conflict' in Vietnam. He says he will enlist in the US
Navy rather than be drafted, as he would feel safer
with his feet on the deck rather than in the jungles.
You want him instead to go with you 'back to
Canada', where his and your grandparents grew up
before coming to the states. He is saying no, he will
not run away.

I'm happy to be able to tell you that he will not be drafted: the country will, in 1970, the year he would be drafted, have the first collective draft, combining youth from ages 18 to 25 in one large lottery, and his birthday will draw a number high enough that many other thousands will go to the war before he would be called. You are both relieved at that, as you are now ready to start a family together.

Your nightly prayer to remain 'happy, healthy, and together' will be rewarded for many years. Some years will be more challenging than others, as the country will continue to struggle with financial recession, gas shortages, inflationary prices, and eventually the demise of the manufacturing jobs that are going to other countries. Your job as a teacher will remain stable.

You will often fear that you will disappoint; you do not disappoint. You will worry about finances, watching other families reap great financial benefits for having chosen other careers; you will never be wealthy in a financial way, but you will always have enough for a home, food, clothing and transportation. It is enough.

In time, you will make decisions with others, for others, and because of others. Some of those decisions will be beneficial for you and for those you love; some will be difficult to make and prove later to have been the wrong decision based on the wrong advice. You will make adjustments, and corrections, and you will live with Rick knowing that decisions about health are never easy, never clear, and you can only make the decisions that you will not look back on with regret. You do this, several times. You learn to trust your instincts.

You will learn that living in the northern latitudes may have affected your health, though in a different way than that of your sisters and brothers. None of them will have the diagnosis that is ahead for you, and so will never make the same decisions about nutrition and physical health that you will have to make. You will stay one step ahead of the curve in those decisions, researching nutrition and medical care and choosing to try and then to stop as you discover what the researchers are finding and slowly revealing to the public. Gradually, you will come to believe that following your own knowledge, instincts, and life lessons will guide you to make the best decisions for you, regardless of what others may suggest in disagreement.

Vitamin D deficiency will be a part of your retirement. Supplementing that and other vitamins will become important to you in your late fifties, but no one will advise you of that, and you will eventually read about it and move in the direction that will benefit you. Be confident and follow your instincts and your knowledge.

I wish I could advise you not to worry, but it is in your nature to worry, to plan, to prepare for the next challenge, and to work hard to overcome each hurdle in your path. Worry seems to work for you.

You will take a quiet advisory role in your sixties, sharing research and findings through something called a blog, where people can stop in and read and make their own decisions about what you have found. And it will be enough. They have to make their own decisions, their own changes, and their own adjustments. You may not be there to see their decisions and their results. You do not have to be there. You have to make your own decisions, and they will have to make theirs.

You will always be wary of what life will place in your path. But you will always be prepared with self-sought knowledge, with determination, and with strength that at times seems heaven-granted.

You will find happiness in realizing that enough is simply that: enough.

11

Choose a Theme Song for the Blog

Today's writing prompt: Imagine your health focus or blog is getting its own theme song... lyrics? Type of music?

The song that comes immediately to mind for me is John Lennon's "Imagine." The lyrics would not change very much from his own: Listen while you read: for those who don't have a copy of Lennon's music, you'll find it free at YouTube.com. Read the lyrics below while listening:

Imagine there's no **heaven**   **illness**
It's easy if you try
No **hell below** us   **pain within**
Above us only sky

Imagine all the people
Living for today
Ahaha...

Imagine there's no **country**   **diagnosis**
It isn't hard to do
Nothing to **kill or die** for   **hurt or cry**
And no **religion** too   **prescription**

Imagine all the people
Living life in peace
You may say I'm a dreamer
But I'm not the only one
I hope some day you'll join us
And the world will be as one

Imagine no **possessions**   **depression**
I wonder if you can
No need for **greed or hunger**   **pills or needles**
A brotherhood of man

Imagine all the people
Sharing all the world
You may say I'm a dreamer
But I'm not the only one
I hope someday you join us
And the world will live as one.

John Lennon was a dreamer, and he advocated a
lifestyle that leaned toward making his dreams
come true. In that sense I am a dreamer, choosing
to believe that good nutrition and exercise will help
me to live the life I choose to live, rather than living
a life focused on injections, medication adjustments,
and fear of degeneration. I would rather do this
naturally, and live as well as I can. I'm grateful to be
able to make this choice.

12

Stream of Consciousness day

Stream of consciousness ... conscientiousness ... thinking about thinking ... metacognition ... what is it I'm thinking of when I'm not thinking on purpose ... I'm not sure ... I think I would be thinking about not thinking, and wondering why I'm trying not to think of something.

The old joke is that when you tell someone not to think of an elephant, that is all they can think of. Asking us to write in a stream of consciousness ... would almost make it impossible to do that, for we're thinking of trying not to think on purpose. Why do I keep coming back to that?

Word association is easier to do ... I wonder if that will come up in a prompt? This seems silly, thinking about not thinking purposely but recording what random thoughts may stray through our conscious selves. I guess I'm not ready yet to live such an unstructured life ... if I'm writing something, it is to be read, either by others, or by myself in another time ... I wouldn't bother to write it otherwise. Even private poetry deserves a re-reading by the author if no one else.

This is not my favorite prompt ... maybe I'm too worried about not doing this right, not being able to write without thinking, or write of thinking.

13

10 Things I Couldn't Live Without

Today's writing prompt is asking me to write about the ten things I couldn't live without. Things. People are not things, so I'll start this list by saying that the people in my life are much more important than the things. I could do without everything as long as I could keep my husband, children and grandchildren in my life. There are many other people in my life who bring me pleasure - friends, colleagues, relatives and acquaintances, but they are not an essential life source for me as my family is. Love is a powerful resource, reciprocal at its best, and devastating if lost.

Love is not a thing ... it's an idea, an emotion, a state of being, a quest, and a gift. I could not live without the love of my family.

Health is not a thing: it is a state of being, but perceived differently by individuals. I have a strong label on my medical folders: multiple sclerosis. It carries with it a prognosis unknown, with the bleakest projections far away on the spectrum from the mildest, benign end. End, you say? There is no end to a spectrum. And if you believe that, then both ends are equally infinite, and the darkest belief is balanced by the brightest.

If this is to be a bucket list of sorts ... the ten things I could not live without ... I really have to play with the word things, because what I could not live without are intangible ideas or states of being. there is nothing tangible on my list:

1.   LOVE: to be loved, and to love in return,

2.   SELF-WORTH: a belief that I can love and be loved

3.   COMPETENCE: being able to provide what I can do to better the states of others

4.   COMPASSION: to receive compassion and to feel compassion for others

5.   UNDERSTANDING: a set of knowledge and an awareness of what that knowledge might provide

6.   APPRECIATION: for those I love, for the world of nature in which we live, for air, food, water and shelter

7.   COURAGE: to face whatever obstacles stand in the way of those I love

8.   WILL: to overcome those obstacles despite whatever personal challenges I feel at the time

9.   SUCCESS: as defined for myself, and as recognized by those I love, and in those I love

10. SELF-CONFIDENCE: to allow myself to speak up for those I love, and for myself.

Are these 'things' that I expect to be given? No. They are emotions, beliefs, values and goals that I have accepted and sought in my life. They are what I have lived, and have tried to model for those I love, that they, too, can live such a life ... where material things have less value, less importance, and are less essential than the way we can live, with whatever we have, wherever we are, and whoever we will be, with and for each other.

Does this list negate the existence or importance of a spiritual belief? Does it neglect homage to a superior being? Does it remove the obligation of duty to a religious belief? Does it place us above a God?

If in reading this list, one is discomforted by the absence of a deity in name, then one is missing all that lies between the lines. Hindus, Taoists and Buddhists recognize the existence of the greatest spirit within ourselves and each other. Their greeting, Namaste, expresses this belief, this recognition, and this humility. Isn't it hubris, you might ask, to assume that the greatest deity resides within us? Humble may be the word ... no one of us is any better, nor any less, than any other of us. "The divine within me recognizes and bows to the divine within you." What a powerful message to share with everyone in your life ... those you love ... those you dislike ... those you fear ... those you feel responsible toward ... Namaste is the great equalizer. It is a word that challenges each of us to be worthy, to be better, to be as loving and compassionate a provider as we may have been taught to believe that God is.

Namaste, my friend. I trust that you understand my writings. They are written from within, with love.

14

Dream Day

Saturday morning, and the day's prompt is to write about my dream day, and whether it has happened yet, and if not, how might I make it happen?

There's a song that came out just about the time that Rick and I had set our wedding date. It was sung by The Sandpipers, and began with the words "Come Saturday Morning, I'm going away with my friend..."

Every little girl's dream day would be her wedding day, and in that sense, I was like any other little girl (although, to confess, there was the matter of believing that Queen Elizabeth's real child (me) had been replaced with a boy, for the sake of the crown, and I dreamed that one day Prince Charles would return, admit the deception, and allow me to assume my rightful place in the castle. But I digress...)

Rick and I had watched the political scene from a distance (we weren't old enough to vote until after our first child was born.) The Vietnam 'conflict' was taking many of our generation away ... some marriages were hastily arranged as a result. But I was a planner, and we were responsible, and we would wait until he'd finished school to marry. We'd been good friends for five years, dating for three, and betrothed for two by the time we were married, and we were quite sure that it was the right thing to do. Others may have thought waiting until the new draft lottery was held would be a wiser choice, but we knew, draft or not, military service or not, we were meant to be married. And so we set the date, and like the young couples of the day, yielded the arrangements and guest list to our parents.

I'd planned to carry lilacs from the bushes on our front lawn; my mother warned me that they would be wilted by May 30th, and they were, so my bouquet was a family prayerbook covered in ivy and stefanotis strands, simple, and humbling. The groomsmen all came on time despite the fact that many had attended their senior prom the night before. The bridal party was dressed in bright spring colors of mint and maize, carrying bouquets of daisies and roses in light whites and yellows tightly gathered, and it looked as though my simple bouquet had been planned that way.

The reception, with a turkey dinner and red wine (which we were not yet old enough, at 20, to drink) was filled with dancing and all the traditional games ... throwing the garter to the single men, and the bouquet to the single young ladies ... clinking the glasses to encourage another kiss for the bride and groom ... dancing with the father of the bride, and the mother of the groom, and then the tin cans tied to the rear bumper, with a printed wedding napkin tucked into the gas cap, to alert all that this was a wedding couple.

It was the day a dream came true, and was followed by yet another soon after, when the draft lottery spared Rick ... and yet again, when our daughter was born a year later ... and many years later when our son was born.

Our most recent dream day was this past Thanksgiving weekend, when, with a generous gift certificate I'd received at my retirement party, we were able to go with our daughter, son, and grandchildren out for a well-appointed brunch by shore of the Atlantic. All of us at the table -not nearly the size it would have taken for all of us in the olden days - being attended by wait staff and being allowed to wander among the buffet tables laden with traditional breakfast items and tea-time treats as well gave me pause to think, and thank.

I am so blessed with love. My life is made up of my dreams come true.

15

Writing with Style

"There is nothing to writing. All you do is sit down at a typewriter and bleed."
-- *Ernest Hemingway*

Well, for centuries writers bled onto paper, then into notebooks, and eventually onto a typewriter's keyboard. The question for today is how do I write?

I've written of this earlier, this awareness that writing with pen and notebook is different than composing on a keyboard; one is not faster than the other for me, though one is definitely more legible.

Years ago I had neat, precise handwriting that flowed beautifully across pages and pages in short time. My thoughts flowed as quickly with my hand; at some times, my brain and my hand would compete, one seemingly yielding to the other. My writing was more sentimental then ... more filled with emotions, happiness, sadness, and yes, anger and resentment.

My writing today is done on a laptop; it is a bit more formal, a bit more reserved, perhaps less expressive and more peaceful in tone. Some of that may be as related to where I am in my life as well as in the change of method. I have less to stress about; I have fewer worries. I am satisfied with the completion of parts of my life, and can look more calmly at what may still be ahead, having weathered all that I've weathered so far.

I used to write about what was still ahead with apprehension, with some fear, and with some prayer. My prayers are now more often of gratitude than of request. My success in life is no longer tied to the vagaries of my students' lives ... my own children are now adults and have experienced some successes, enough to feel confident in going ahead. My husband and I are almost out of the mortgaged years, and while we don't have extra money for retirement vacations, we have a home where we are both happy, I with my sewing machine, computer and greenhouse, and he with his workshop, tools, and customers. We both feel close enough to the finish line of life to realize that we will at least approach it together, and that if we cross it at separate times, the one left behind will be there with happy, contented memories.

Is catastrophic illness still ahead of us? Possibly. Will our children find a way to cope with and survive that part of the journey with us? Yes. Will they be in unison at the time? Perhaps, perhaps not. Will they be able to look at how our generation handled that, and choose to follow or digress from the modeled path? Yes, certainly. Will they, too, be able to make the choices that will not leave them in regret later? Yes. Will they define regret or satisfaction in their own terms, in their own circumstances, in their own time? No doubt. Will it be the same as ours was? We will not know that ... but we trust that they will do what is right for them, and for us.

Would I have written that differently in a notebook? At the time I wrote in notebooks, yes, certainly, for all of those challenges were yet ahead of me, of us. It is not just the ability to write legibly that I have lost to the years and to the diagnosis of ... whatever it is I have ... Multiple Sclerosis or Parkinson's Disease. I have lost so much more. I have lost the fear of not measuring up in terms and decisions of responsibility. I have lost the pressing schedule of teaching every day in a classroom of students who might be experiencing their own trials. I have lost the need to work through pain, fatigue, and worry.

I have gained a measure of peace, and believe in increased peace ahead. Past fears and worries will fade in memory, in time. Do I want them to be unseen and forgotten entirely - no, I want my children and grandchildren to know that it was not easy, it was not totally surpassed, it was approached with fear, but also with love, and it was, in its own time, finished. And their challenges yet ahead will be, too, one day. And so I write, or type, or enter ... for them, as much as for me.

16

Open a book and write!

Today's Health Awareness writing prompt is: open a
book, see a phrase, and write about it for 15
minutes.

I opened a book by Robert Fulgham, found on my
daughter's bookshelf. The phrase I read is:"... it can
always be worse than the list"

Of course, my first thought is, what list? But that
would take me away from the intent of the prompt.
So instead, I will write about a list that I have been
following all week while staying at her house.

It's a list of morning chores: after getting the kids'
morning needs met so that they are ready on time
for the high school bus, there are the animals to care
for: not many, but their needs are very different.

The dog has an egg beat into his morning dry food,
so his bowl must first be washed. As his water bowl
has to be filled anyway, I wash that, too. I stir his
egg in his empty bowl, then add a scoop of dog food,
then stir it into the egg. He sits patiently at my feet
as I do this. I wash his water bowl then, and half fill
it, and put both bowls on the floor. If there are
leftovers of the kids' toast or bagels (not usually) I'll
add that to his food, too.

Then the fish - there are only two, and they don't
need much. A small pinch of flaked fish food and a

small pinch of freeze-dried blood worms (which don't look like worms at all.) Then top off the water in their tank, and watch them find the food. The sucker fish actually turns on his back and skims along just underneath the surface of the water, scooping up the flakes that are floating there, as though he were cleaning them from the sides of the tank. And the small black shark with the pointed nose and two tiny whiskers darts around the tanks foliage, snatching for the blood worms, and rejecting the flakes. To each his own.

Last on the pet list is the family's bird, a cockatiel (I may have that name wrong) who greets me each morning when I remove his cage cover with a seductive whistle. I remove, wash and refill his water, and then dump the remainders of his seeds (mostly empty husks) and fill it with new seed. If I remember, I'll give him a slice of peeled apple, or a bit of fresh lettuce. He talks in chirps to me as I'm doing it, interspersing his language with whistles he has learned. I've taught him to imitate the sound of a cardinal, and he does that quite well. He somewhere learned how to imitate a donkey, and a chirp that sounds very much like 'hurry up,' which gets me moving or calls me back to finish whatever I'd forgotten. And yes, I have to agree with Robert Fulgham: it could always be worse than the list: it could be many more animals, with pens that need to be cleaned out. Or it could be many more animals and not enough food to share. It can always be worse.

The animals have been wonderful company with me this week - the dog curls up in bed at night with me, the bird greets me flirtatiously each morning, and the fish are mesmerizing to watch as they share the tank gracefully. When the kids come home from school, there are more lists of reminders, but they, too, are enjoyable and loving.

Life could certainly be worse than it is! I've had a wonderful two weeks with them all.

17
What five people would you invite to a dinner party, and why?

I have to expect that my immediate family (husband, daughter and companion, son and companion, and grandchildren) would already be at the table with me. And, we always set an extra place. So here are my six guests:
In that case, I would like to invite Hillary Clinton (accompanied by her husband, Bill), in order to thank her for her service to our country as Secretary of State in such difficult years.
I would next want to invite Barack Obama and his wife, and two daughters. I would want to thank them for the decision to stay at the White House at great personal expense, and for the benefit their presence gives to the rest of America.
These six people are currently in the position to advocate for improved health care for all Americans, and are currently receiving top notch medical care

for themselves. Their futures are assured by earned pensions, and their safety is in good hands with the secret service protection no matter where they are in the world.

All six of them have every reason to want to sit together at the same table; I would love to have my family break bread and have a chance to talk freely with each of them.

As a teacher, I would want to engage the Obama daughters in a conversation about how they are developing their own social and political beliefs, and how the move to Washington may have affected those. My own grandchildren would no doubt have some comments to share about attending public high school in a state widely impacted by the economic decline.

As a retired teacher whose pension was affected by a premature retirement caused by a diagnosis and treatment that weakened me both physically and emotionally, I would want both Hillary and Barack to hear my limited economic rewards for thirty years of dedicated, 'highly qualified' teaching. I would want my son to have a chance to explain to them that though he works more than forty hours through multiple positions as a highly skilled public servant he is not yet entitled to quality health insurance. I would want my daughter to have an opportunity to ask both of them how they are working to improve the long-term economic planning to benefit her children. I would want my husband to have a chance to point out that his years of unpaid elder care have limited his maximum earnings towards pension and social security benefits.

I would like to give our dinner guests a healthy menu, one which would feature vegetables, grains, clear filtered water and fresh fruit for dessert. I would like to host this dinner during cold winter weather, using our wood stove to supplement the oil furnace that we really cannot afford to turn higher. While the stove would keep them comfortable, they would see that carrying in the wood and maintaining the fire and the area surrounding the stove would take energy and attention, more so than simply turning a thermostat higher.

I would ask our guests to bow their head for a moment of silence, meditation or prayer, just as I did with my colleagues for thirty years of public education. And I would teach them the Pledge of Allegiance in American Sign Language, explaining the meaning so evidently attached to each word's sign. And then, after dinner, I would offer a simple grace expressing thankfulness for the healthy food and good company shared.

18

*What is a **lesson** you learned the hard way?*

Sometimes we let our ego get in the way of logic. After trying to meet the requirements of Smashwords' e-pub format and failing repeatedly, you would think I could have allowed myself to seek help ... well, I did seek help - I asked my son to take a look at the mess I had made at the time of the first failure ... the helpful directions at Smashwords were highly technical in language ... and as my son wasn't there when I made the errors, he couldn't help me puzzle out the solution.

I tried again. I tried a third time. I read the difficult guidelines over and over, trying to absorb by osmosis their meaning. As best I could tell, my computer was unable to leave Microsoft Office and work solely in Word, and so my file was continually rejected.

Only when I learned that other authors left the formatting woes to folks who offered to work with their files for a nominal fee (in my case, offers ranged between twenty and fifty dollars) did I let myself seek that help.

The first formatter advertised his rates as between twenty-five and fifty, and when he learned that my book had twenty chapters he quoted at the high end but advised that his work was guaranteed and would be completed within 72 hours. I said thank you very much, but I can't afford that right now.

Discouraged, I went back to the other authors, and asked what they thought of the offer. One gave me the name of another formatter on the list, someone who had done the work slowly and carefully and for less money. I contacted that person, sent her my file, and she agreed that she could do it in a matter of two weeks. She sent me the completed file last night.

But in transferring it from my email to my desktop, and then on to Smashwords, the issue of Works to Word again reared its head. Her file was apparently corrupted by the process. She had an answer, though, and sent the file again through something called Wetransfer.com. I was able to save directly from the email without opening the document, and forwarded it on successfully to Smashwords.

Once again, though, Smashwords rejected my

submission, saying that the jpeg cover image was too small. I had encountered that problem before, when I submit the cover for a Rack Card order with Vistaprint. I had enlarged it to their required size, but it became 'pixilated' and the result was blurry. I ordered it anyway, not expecting perfection and happy to settle with what I had. Smashwords wasn't of a like mind. They don't settle.

The formatter helped me again, this time in somehow enlarging the jpeg without blurring the image, bless her.

What does this teach me about myself, and how do I connect this to health? A year ago, when I was trying to submit my first book to Smashwords, I was in a different place, emotionally. I was continually butting my head against the proverbial brick wall, seeing no way around or over it. Calmer now, I am often remembering my dad's advice ... to turn to a new direction that will benefit others as well as myself.

Hiring someone to do the work for me made sense, just as it makes sense for other authors to hire me to improve their drafts through proofreading or editing. We cannot all be good at everything; knowing that, and choosing to do what we are good at, is a privilege adults have. Schools expect students to succeed in every subject - which is why Edison, Einstein and other highly intelligent creative thinkers do better learning in their own smaller sphere. The cartoon that so eloquently addresses this issue is one that shows a rabbit, a bear, a turtle, a fish and some other creature. They are all asked to demonstrate proficiency in climbing a tree. Point made.

19

Choose a mascot: real, fictional or mythical, for your condition.

If you read my blog yesterday, you read a book review of **Birth of the Phoenix**, by Harriett B. Varney Miller. And in reading and reviewing the book, I was reacquainted with the symbolism of the phoenix, the bird that weakens and dies in a smoldering heap of ash, and then rises, whole and new and better than before. What better 'mascot' to have, what better symbol, than this mythical bird? In the book, she represented the strength of battered women who have the opportunity to remake their lives.

With MS, it is easy to first be defeated by the prognosis that accompanies the diagnosis. Multiple Sclerosis is a progressive, degenerative disease that can attack any body function, as it rests within the central nervous system, potentially affecting any combination of nerves that conduct message from the brain through the spinal column to all body parts. Not only can it affect mobility, sight, speech, touch, hearing, taste or smell; it can also affect memory, thought processes, the ability to logically organize thought, plan, and strategize with other higher order thinking skills. And so, it affects not only your life, but the lives of all who care for you, and are cared for by you. It affects your career, your co-workers, and those you may serve in a career: students, patients, clients, and customers who are depending on you for a service such as teaching, nursing, advocacy and other careers.

Initially, the doctor who has the answers is seen as delivering a definitive diagnosis and prescription. The prescription comes with a vague and limited suggestion of a slowing of the progression. You have a choice at this point to reject, accept, or postpone acceptance of this diagnosis. Yet, most people see doctors as infallible, and diagnoses as black and white. In time, you might realize that something doesn't fit, and you may rethink your agreement or rejection.

If you are like me, you may experience a complete deterioration of your life plans and goals, given the limitations that impose themselves on your functioning in the way you are used to functioning. If you are as lucky as I, you have friends and family who will support you through this dark period, and help you to remember that it is your life, and your choice as to whether to agree or disagree with the treatment.

I was able to rise from the ash pile of my former self and create a new me, and begin in a new direction. No longer could I remember one hundred students names at a time. No longer could I organize their individual styles, strengths, weaknesses and needs in my mind, and meet each one where they needed to be met. No longer could I sit at a meeting table with anxious parents seeking advice based on careful observation. No longer could I be a confident public school teacher.

While struggling with those losses, I was still functioning, despite the odd symptoms that come with multiple sclerosis. I realized that having agreed to the daily injections, I had accepted the diagnosis despite my consistent and strong belief that this was not MS but something else, something more familiar. I understood then that continuing for four and a half years with injections that troubled me physically, emotionally and economically had brought me down into a depression that deepened by the day, week and month.

And when I could see that clearly... when I could make my decision to stop pretending to agree... when I could stop trying to look like I did have MS and stop injecting something that had the power to affect every nerve in my body, I stopped.

And then I became: I became who I am today, with the strength and confidence of my old self restored, and I arose from the ashes of my aberrant, temporary, indelibly-labeled-with-MS-self. The rejection of the prescription and cessation of injections restored my daily independence. The release from the nightly pain following each injection allowed me to fall asleep at peace with myself, having escaped the unrelenting reminder of this diagnosis. With the help of an antidepressant medication and talk therapy with a psychologist, I began living again, not just existing, and more than just surviving.

Who I am today is a writer, an author, a thinker, an observer, a recorder, and a self-marketer. I am happy with what I have become, and I accept what I've had to leave behind. Phoenix is better with each new rebirth. I have that to look forward to, whenever it may occur yet again.

20

The Things We Forget

I used to need a list to remember everything I
needed to take with me when I left the house at 6:30
in the morning ... I taped the list to the frame of the
back door, so that I would see it as I left. Here is the
list:

Iron turned off
Coffee turned off
computer bag
school bag
cell phone
travel cup of coffee
lunch bag
lights off
door locked

Those were the things that were necessary for me to
leave town with peace of mind, knowing I would not
have to turn around to go back for one or two of
them if forgotten. These were in the years when Rob
was in college, Rick was working an earlier day than
I, and I was leaving the house last.

These were the years after my parents had passed,
and before my diagnosis of RRMS had begun. Our
lives had settled down somewhat, but my memory
of last minute details was weakening. Evenings
extended into late nights with paperwork taking
more time and energy each night ... correcting
essays was becoming more difficult, recording
scores on a computerized spreadsheet with tiny

squares and failing eyesight ... age was taking its toll as well.

But during my last few years at school, Rick was home with me in the morning, and he did his best to be sure that I had all that I'd need for the day each morning. Still, the list stayed taped in place.

Now retired, I don't have to rush anywhere. I don't have to leave and lock a door behind me, worrying that I'm forgetting something. I can sleep in most mornings. I have no papers to correct, no scores to record, no meetings to remember and no worries about deadlines.

Rick and I are almost always together now. We are back to sharing one vehicle. We double-check each other and laugh when we've both forgotten something. But the list is still taped to the back door frame ~ a reminder that the good old days are behind us now, and we are living our happily ever after, together, and safe.

21

Write a memory, in third person, using all sensory references:

This is a memory of 22 years ago, when Rob was still a toddler, his mother yet undiagnosed.

The two were smiling as she drove along the highway, he in his car seat beside her, with the radio playing oldies. Dad was not with them, as he was caring for Gram in those days, and late afternoon was a time when he was needed to read her the mail, pay whichever bills had come in, and check to see that she had what was needed for supper.

As they took the ramp exiting the highway, her son began watching traffic with her.
"There's a dump truck, Mum ... and that's a ... that's a brown truck."
"Can you read the letters on that truck, Rob?" she asked him, downshifting as they came to the end of the ramp and the bright red stop sign, shining in the

afternoon sun.

"It's U P S, Mum. I don't know what that says. But the red sign says stop!"

She did stop, and looked to the left, then pulled out carefully into the traffic. The ride from the highway to the shore was busy with commuters who lived year round at the beach and were anxious to get home before the sun set, as the reflective glow on the eastern shore was going to be spectacular.

They were following the brown truck now, until it turned right into a busy shopping plaza. The traffic lights ahead were just turning yellow, and then red, and they stopped again. Rob had settled back in his car seat, and was watching the lights. As soon as the green light lit, he said "That means go, Mum. Why are we still stopped?"

Before she could answer, traffic began to move, and she eased into the left lane as they approached the turn toward the beach. Heading north, the scenery changed dramatically from the commercial area to a residential one, with large houses built to the left of the road, and a sea wall and dunes off to the right. Rob watched out his window, and she slowed as she approached the spot where they would find a jetty and tide pools. The parking lot ahead was still fairly empty as the temperature was brisk; not many came out to enjoy the sea in late winter, but then was when she found it most beautiful.

They pulled in diagonally to a space near the opening in the sea wall, and took the kite out from behind the seat. Standing beside his door, she made sure his knitted hat was pulled down over his ears, his jacket was zipped up over his scarf, and his mittens were tucked into the cuffs of his sleeves. Then she lifted him down to the pavement, and let him climb up onto the wall. He began to walk carefully along the top, with his mother walking alongside him. She stepped through the opening and met him on the sandy side, and lifted him down onto the still-frozen sand.

Rob held the kite and she unrolled the reel of string, walking away from him but still tethered by the kite. His eyes squinted in the wind, and he watched her for their signal. When he saw her lift the reel high over her head, he gave the open kite a push up over his, and she began to pump the string. Gradually the kite lifted, tilting crazily side to side until it had enough height to rise steadily upward on the south wind. Rob ran toward his mother; together they held the reel, his mittened hands within her cold fingers, working together to guide the kite into the face of the wind. The seagulls began squawking and squealing as the multicolored diamond with the long flapping tale hovered over the tide pools, interrupting their foraging. They were backed up far enough now that Rob could climb over the rocks and look down into the tide pools, searching for urchins with their sturdy, bristly covering. Finding even the discarded shell of one would be a treasure, but none were to be found this time. Coming back to his mother, they both leaned against the seawall and watched the reflection over the water of the sun setting behind them.

Pink turned to lilac, and then lavender, and then violet. "We better hurry - the bugs will be out soon," she said to him. She began reeling in the kite slowly, careful not to pull so hard against the wind that the string would break. Rob watched as it jerked and bobbed over the water, and when it lowered enough and was back over wet sand he ran toward the sea to catch it's landing.

They ran together back toward the truck, and she lifted him again onto the wall and passed through the opening. He hopped down to the pavement, and stood by the door as she wrapped the kite back into a narrow twist and tucked it behind the seat. Lifting him up and buckling him in, she saw the first of the small flies landing on the sun-warmed windshield. She hurried over to her door, got in, and looked across the seat at Rob, who was counting the flies as they arrived.

"Six, seven ... we beat them here, Mum." They continued to gather, seeking the warmth of the still warm engine.

"Will dad be home when we get there?" She nodded, and reached over to pull his mittens off. He reached up to his head and pushed the hat off his forehead. Starting the engine, they waited a few more minutes, watching the violet sky turn to dark purple, navy blue, and then looked for stars ... but saw none.

"Where is Venus, Mum?" he asked, puzzled.

"We'll see her when we get back on the highway. She's in the south-west, waiting for us. There's no cloud cover tonight; it's going to be very cold when we get home."

"And the moon will be with Venus? And Dad will be at home, right? And he will make a fire in the wood stove, right?"

"Right," she said, driving carefully toward the highway, and home.

ABOUT THE AUTHOR

Terry Crawford Palardy took 'early' retirement after thirty years in public classrooms, teaching all content areas grades 1 through 8, in both general and special education classrooms. She attended five colleges earning several honors, and taught graduate courses in education as an adjunct faculty member for Lesley University in Cambridge.

After retiring, she gathered up samples of her writing and composed several books, with topics of education, poetry, small town life and chronic illnesses. She then began writing a new mystery series, based on characters much like herself and her husband, Rick, but projected forward fifteen years and living in their eighties, with a quilt shop and wooden gift shop. All of her books can be found at her web store: www.TerryCrawfordPalardy.com. They are also available at Amazon.com, and at Smashwords.com.

A year after posting these Health Blog entries, Terry opened her own quilt/fabric shop, sharing the space of Rick's Wooden Toy and Gift Shop, and continues today to meet the most heart-warming members of the community of quilters and needle workers.

With both children grown and grandchildren in college, Terry and Rick are living their happily ever after years together, and their shops bring them much joy, which they share freely with all who visit them.

www.ingramcontent.com/pod-product-compliance
Lightning Source LLC
Chambersburg PA
CBHW062056280526
45788CB00003B/1242